Can five ancient Tibetan rites really make you look and feel years younger? Read what others are saying . . .

Here are actual quotes from letters and notes sent in by readers:

■ "I felt the difference after the *first* day! Now into my 4th week, I'm looking younger and feeling more vitality every day."—Dolores H., Chelan, WA

■ "After just 5 weeks, lines, crows-feet and age spots are disappearing. And here's the fun part: Though I'm 40 years old and looked every year of it, people now guess that I'm 35, 29, or even 26 years young. Yes, the 5 rites do work. All you have to do is try them, and in a little while you can be a beautiful person again. Bless you. I sincerely thank you for the gift of youth."—Barbara Crockett, Las Vegas, NV

Look Younger

■ "Having performed the 5 rites for over a year, I am looking much younger. . . some say 15 years younger. My weak ankles have strengthened and my posture has improved. My body is more flexible and nimble."
— La Mae Lemkuil, Oostburg, WI

■ "I not only feel younger, but am told by people who know my age (73) that I look and act 20 years younger. My doctor, who is 58, complained that although he jogs 15 to 20 miles per week, I look younger than he does. I recommend this book to anyone who wants to halt the aging process."—Jack Smith, Grass Valley, CA

■ "I was amazed at what my friends said after I had applied the 5 rites for 3 months. They wanted to know why I was looking so much younger than before — some said 15 years younger. I am really excited that such a thing as the 'Fountain of Youth' does truly exist."
—Bernard Davis, Liberty, NY

Feel Younger

■ "Recently a friend of mine began to look much younger, and his full gray beard began to turn a lovely shade of brown. Upon questioning he told me about the Fountain of Youth book. Since I started doing the 5 rites, here's what's happened to me: My insomnia and eczema have disappeared completely. My hot flashes said goodbye (I'm 53). After 25 years of bifocals, I no longer need glasses. And my eyes have turned a lovely shade of blue, like 25 years ago. I feel like I'm 16 again, but I'm really going to miss my lovely silver hair. It's the only thing I like about being older."
—Ida Schultz, Salt Lake City, UT

■ "After about 3 months of doing the 5 rites, many people began telling me I was looking much younger, and upon looking in the mirror, I had to agree with them. When they wanted to know what I was doing, I told them about the Fountain of Youth book which they subsequently purchased. Now that they have been doing the 5 rites for a while, they are looking younger too."
—Charles Tepper, Brooklyn, NY

New Hair Growth

■ "For a while, my hair was thinning and coming out. Now, it is growing in again and becoming thicker."
—Henry Van Olst, Hawthorne, NJ

■ "When my doctor's family saw me after about 5 years, they said, 'What have you done? We know you're 75, but you look and act about 35 or 40. Your hair is no longer white and balding, but gray and thick. Tell us your secret.' I showed them my Fountain of Youth book, and since they are good friends of many years, I lent it to them. Needless to say, I'll never see that book again."
—H.B. McCauley, Tularosa, NM

■ "When I began the rites my beard & mustache were so gray and my skin so pale, I looked like the ghost of my grandfather. Now my body has a good tone & complexion, and my beard and mustache has gradually changed color until it is nearly black. Also, I can read fine print, something I could never do before."
—Chas. Hamilton, Thousand Oaks, CA

Amazing Energy

■ "I've been working pretty intensively at self-improvement methods for almost 15 years, but I *NEVER* felt anything quite as good as the 5 rites... After the third week I began to feel the most amazing and incredible increase in energy and vitality. It was truly dramatic and astounding!"
—Joe Alexander, Fayetteville, AR

■ "Although I have been practicing the 5 rites only a few weeks, my vitality has increased tremendously. It may sound far fetched, but my awareness is also much more acute. I'm elated!" —Myra C., Yakima, WA

■ "I recommended your book to several patients who later came back with glowing reports. So, I began doing the 5 rites myself 3 weeks ago. After about 9 days I felt a great increase in strength and endurance. I was able to climb stairs with heavy packages, without any strain. A nutritionist I recently met told me he performed the 5 rites for 4 months and became much stronger, even though he was athletic for years and lifted weights regularly. His friends told him he had become younger looking. I have great confidence in your book, and intend to go all the way with it."
—Dr. Stanley S. Bass, D.C., Ph.C., Brooklyn, NY

Better Memory

■ "My memory was getting so bad I was ashamed. Now, after using the 'rites' daily for 2 months, I seem to be getting clarity of mind, and much, much more energy. My friends notice the change too. I am truly thankful that at age 62 I am 'youthing' instead of aging."
—Adeline Neveu, Yakima, WA

■ "At age 83 I had lost all interest in life. I was thinking of putting myself in a home, and didn't think I would live much longer. Then, I discovered your book about the 5 rites. I have been doing them only a short time, but already my memory has improved 50%, and I feel so much more alive. Everyone tells me I am looking younger all the time. Thanks to the 5 rites, I am a completely different person now, and am continuing to improve. Everyone should read this book." —E.B.K. Miller, Buxton, NC

■ "This comes from what was a

physical wreck a few months ago. I had only enough energy to lace one shoe, and then I had to rest. Now I can lift a hundred pounds and walk away with it. This is the greatest book I've ever read in my life."

—L.H. Chambers, Bainville, MT

■ "I must tell you that I have never before experienced such a wonderful sense of well-being, joy and harmony, strength and stamina. It is really amazing, because I am a great-grandmother of 74!...P.S. I seem to need fewer hours of sleep, and because I am more relaxed, I sleep more deeply."

—Jytte Fyrst, Oslo, Norway

Energy, Lasting Power

■ "I used to come home from work feeling absolutely exhausted—even on weekends after getting plenty of sleep. Since doing the rites, I'm always alert and full of energy. This past summer I had more energy than anyone else on my softball team. The change has been absolutely unbelievable."

—Linda Felder, Silver Spring, MD

■ "I used to drag myself half asleep to class in the morning. After I do the rites, though, I feel refreshed and alert, even looking forward to my studies. Also, I've been working out for quite some time with only mediocre results. Since starting the rites I notice a dramatic improvement in my performance and an increase in how much I can lift. I'm not sure I buy the metaphysical explanation, but I am sure that the 5 Rites work—Thank You!"

—Mark Perkins, Lansing, MI

■ "I immediately noticed a change in my energy and feeling of well-being. My days flow better, and I have more lasting power at my job. This is true only when I do the 5 rites."

—A Satisfied Participant, Age 48

Fat & Flab Vanish

■ "My body, which was flabby, is quickly becoming firm and supple — and it's been only 11 weeks since I began the 5 rites. What is even more amazing is the sensation of control. My body feels as light and responsive as it did in my twenties. Also, I feel much more energetic and cheerful. My friend says the rites help one tune into the universal source of well being and eliminate all negativity."

—Assya Humesky, Ann Arbor, MI

■ "With the 5 rites I am building muscle and dropping fatty tissue. I feel much better now, and am expecting even more improvement soon. I recommend this book very highly to everyone."

—Charles Knower, Los Angeles, CA

■ "Ten days ago I tried on my sister's dress, and the waist was so tight it looked terrible on me. Yesterday, I tried it on again, and it fit beautifully. It's hard to believe that my body shape has improved so much in such a short time, but it has. Also, I have greater stamina. I can work more and bounce back from tiredness much better and faster."

—Ruth O., Alpine, TX

■ "The skin on my arms has tightened enough so that no flab is visible. I recommend the 5 rites to anyone. Just do them with an open mind, and watch the results."

—V.T., Placerville, CA

■ "A vertebra, my hipbone, and a kneecap have gone back into place spontaneously. After years of being dependent on chiropractors, you can imagine how overjoyed I am feeling."

—Bonita Z., Phoenix, AZ

Arthritis Relief

■ After doing the rites regularly for 6 months, my arthritis is gone from both knees, and I come from an arthritic family. I'm so glad I stumbled onto the Colonel's book last year."

—Fred Schmidt, Tavares, FL

■ "After 10 days I noticed that the arthritis disappeared from my fingers. Also, my hair is growing dark in front where I had all white. I feel more vitality too."

—Helena Sutherland, San Anselmo, CA

■ "My feet were swollen for 2 years. I consulted an M.D., a D.O., and 2 foot specialists, and none could help. After doing the 5 Rites one week, the swelling disappeared. Then, within 2 months I lost 5 pounds without changing my diet."

—Don Starkman, Philmath, OR

Sinus Help

■ "Curing years of sinus headaches was my motivation for ordering your book. The day it arrived I began the rites, and I haven't had a sinus headache since. This is a miracle in Virginia, as so many people suffer from sinus problems here."

—Helga Vorda, Reston, VA

■ "No more waking up with one nostril plugged in the morning. My sinus is slowly clearing up. It was unpleasant to say the least."

—Ron McIntosh, Eden, NY

■ "When I started the 5 Rites, my sinus immediately cleared up. My sense of smell is very much sharper than it was before, and my hearing has improved."

—Wm V. Marsh, Randall, VT

■ "Years ago, acute sinusitis caused me to lose my sense of smell. Since starting the 5 rites, my sense of smell has returned. Words cannot describe the thanks I feel."

—Carol M., Tucson, AZ

■ "The results are truly amazing. I now enjoy my sports of golf and tennis without experiencing any soreness whatsoever. I can also do my yard work without pain or muscle soreness. My actual age is 69, but I feel like I'm 45 or 50."

—William Bond, Golden, CO

Pain Relief

■ "I've had a backache for 37 years & after the first day of doing the 5 rites it was gone entirely."

—Kathy Logan, Los Gatos, CA

■ "Due to an old injury, I experienced pain in my left knee for 38 years. Since starting the 5 rites a year ago, my left knee has been as good as my right knee. I can now twist and turn without any discomfort. Also, when I started the 5 rites, a severe shoulder and arm pain left me, and has never returned."

—Charles Pabis, Fayette City, PA

■ "For over 6 months I had severe pain in my legs. I had to take 2 pain pills to get to work, then 2 to get home. After 2 weeks of doing the rites, the pain disappeared. Now, 30 days later, I can work & play all day & night without pills. The rites do work. You may add my name to your list of happy people."

—Wm. T. Spencer, D.C., St. Paul, MN

■ "My lower back problem is much

better now, and I seldom get pain there anymore."

—Thomas H. Hentz, Ellensburg, WA

■ "A serious spinal injury left me disabled and in extreme pain for 5 years. I even considered ending my life until I read your book. Now, thanks to the 5 rites, the pain is relieved, I can walk again, and I have even been able to find work as a pre-school teacher."

—Lynna Turnbow, Reno, NV

■ "I really enjoy the Fountain of Youth book and it has helped me improve my thyroid condition. For almost 25 years I took .3 mg of synthroid, and now I need only .1 mg. When the doctor says he can't believe it is the 5 rites, I just smile."

—Kathy Hernandez, Marina Del Rey, CA

Better Digestion

■ "As I do the 5 rites, I can feel my digestion improving. Also, my head feels clearer. *The Fountain of Youth* is a fascinating book."

—Arthur I., Philadelphia, PA

■ "I have proof that the 5 rites work. A couple of weeks after starting them, my ulcers healed almost completely."—Harriette B., Phoenix, AZ

■ "I haven't tried the 5 rites yet, but I have followed the book's dietary recommendations with very noticeable results. I just look younger and better. Every time I go out in public, someone compliments me on my appearance. I seem to eat less food, and have no false appetite for junk foods. I gave copies of the book to friends. When I saw one recently she looked much better also."

—Frances M. Turner, Los Angeles, CA

Never Felt Better

■ "Since I was introduced to the 5 rites, I have not missed a day, and I have never felt better in my life."

—J.R. Watzke, Waunakee, WI

■ "After 2 days I could actually see results. As time goes by, I am seeing further startling improvement. I have purchased a lot of health books, and although they are good ones, nothing has helped me so much in such a short time as your book. I fully consider it an answer to my prayers." —Ruth S., Kansas City, MO

■ "This is one of the best books I know about at this time. I wish all the good people in the world knew about it."

—Nina Stewart, Gloucester, MA

■ "Thank you for publishing this wonderful book. Once I started to read it, I couldn't put it down . . . P.S. I'm 77 and have been looking for a book like this all my life!"

—Evelyn Sugden, Allentown, PA

Ancient Secret
of the
Fountain of Youth

New Revised Edition of a Book by

Peter Kelder

HARBOR PRESS, Inc.

Gig Harbor, Washington

Library of Congress Cataloging-in-Publication Data

Kelder, Peter.
    Ancient secret of the fountain of youth.
    Rev. ed. of: The eye of revelation. c1939
    1. Exercise. 2. Longevity. 3. Rejuvenation.
4. Medicine, Tibetan. I. Kelder, Peter. Eye of
revelation. II. Title.
RA781.K36   1985   613.7'1   85-30517
ISBN 0-936197-25-0

Important Notice:

The author of this book is not a medical doctor, and the ideas, positions and statements contained herein may in some cases conflict with orthodox, mainstream medical opinion. The exercises and dietary measures outlined in this book are not suitable for everyone, and under certain circumstances they could lead to injury. You should not attempt self-diagnosis, and you should not embark upon any exercise program, dietary regimen or self-treatment of any kind without qualified medical supervision. Nothing in this book should be construed as a promise of benefits or of results to be achieved. The publisher, its editors and its employees disclaim any liability, loss or risk incurred directly or indirectly as a result of the use and application of any of the contents of this book.

Printed in the United States of America

20

Published by:
Harbor Press, Inc.
P.O. Box 1656
Gig Harbor, WA 98335

Foreword

This wonderfully simple little book is not for everyone. You should read it only if you can accept the preposterous notion that aging can be reversed. You should read it only if you dare believe that the "Fountain of Youth" does truly exist. If you stubbornly cling to the prevailing idea that such things are impossible, reading this book will be a waste of your time. If, on the other hand, you can accept that the "impossible" is really within your grasp, then you are in store for rewards in abundance.

As far as I know, Peter Kelder's book is the only written source of the priceless information it reveals: five ancient Tibetan rites which hold the key to lasting youth, health, and vitality. For thousands of years these seemingly magical rites were shrouded in secrecy in remote Himalayan monasteries. The five rites were first brought to the attention of the Western world in the original edition of Mr. Kelder's book, published almost 50 years ago. Since that time, the book and its extraordinary wealth of information have been largely lost and forgotten. The purpose of this new, revised edition is to bring Mr. Kelder's message back before the public in hope that large numbers of people will be influenced and helped by it.

It is impossible to say whether Mr. Kelder's story of Colonel Bradford is based on fact, fiction, or a blend of the two. But the validity of his message is beyond question. My own experience, as well as letters and notes from readers throughout the world, proves to my complete satisfaction that the five rites do really work! I cannot promise that the rites will erase 50 years from your age, transform you overnight, or make you live to 125. But I do know that they can help anyone to look and feel years younger, and to gain a greater sense of well-being. If you perform the rites daily, you should begin to notice results in 30 days or less. In about ten weeks, you'll probably start to see more substantial benefits. Whatever the pace of your progress, it's always a thrilling moment when friends actually begin to comment that you are looking younger and healthier.

If the five rites really work, the big question is *how?* How could simple exercises have such a profound effect on the body's aging process? It is interesting to note that Mr. Kelder's explanation, which you are about to read, does find some support in recent scientific advancements. Kirlian photography, which shows the body surrounded by an invisible electrical field or "aura," does indeed suggest that we are "fed" by some form of energy that permeates the universe. It is also true that the Kirlian aura of a young, healthy person is different from that of an aging, unhealthy person.

For thousands of years Eastern mystics have maintained that the body has seven principal energy centers corresponding to the seven endocrine glands. The hormones produced by these glands regulate all of our bodily functions. Medical research has recently uncovered convincing evidence that even the aging process is hormone regulated. It appears that the pituitary gland begins producing a "death hormone" at the onset of puberty. This "death hormone" apparently interferes with the ability of cells to utilize beneficial hormones, such as growth hormone. As a result, our cells and organs gradually deteriorate, and finally die. In other words, the aging process takes its toll.

If the five rites do indeed normalize imbalance in the

body's seven energy centers, as Mr. Kelder maintains, perhaps as a consequence hormonal imbalance is normalized also. This could make it possible for our cells to replicate and prosper as they did when we were very young. We could indeed see and feel ourselves growing "younger" day by day.

You may agree or disagree with this point of view. And as you read this book you will find many more points to agree or disagree with. But this is important: Do not allow disagreements to distract you from the book's central issue — the benefits earned by performing the five rites. There is only one way to find out whether the five rites will work for you, and that is to *try them*. Try them and give them a fair chance to succeed.

As with any reward, benefits will come only as a result of your effort. You must be willing to invest a small amount of time and energy to perform the five rites on a daily basis. If after a few weeks you lose interest and perform them only occasionally, don't expect the very best results. Fortunately, most people find the daily routine of performing the five rites not only easy, but also enjoyable.

As you read this book and begin putting the five rites to work for yourself, please keep two things in mind. First, know that you are a wonderfully special person who can see beyond the limited thoughts and opinions of others. If you weren't, this book would not have attracted your attention. Second, know that you deserve to have your most cherished desires fulfilled, even the desire for renewed youth and vitality. Those who deep down inside see themselves as unworthy and undeserving are the ones who seem to never share in life's rewards.

When you hold yourself in high esteem, and when you know that you are worthy of the very best that life can offer, what you are really doing is *loving yourself.* Self-love enables you to feel good about who and what you are, and this greatly speeds the renewal process.

Those who dislike themselves or see themselves as inadequate carry a burden that can only accelerate the ravages of old age and ill health. Those who enrich themselves with the treasure of self-love make all things possible.

—Editor

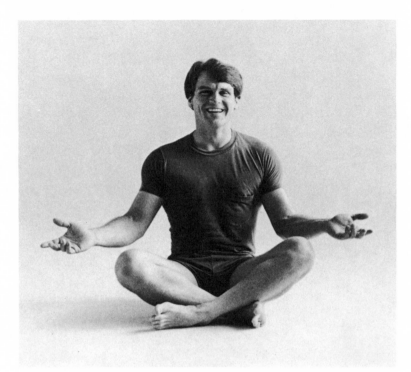

Ancient Secret
of the
Fountain of Youth

Part One

One afternoon some years ago, I was sitting in the park reading the afternoon paper, when an elderly gentleman walked up and seated himself alongside me. Appearing to be in his late sixties, he was gray and balding, his shoulders drooped, and he leaned on a cane as he walked. Little did I know that from that moment, the whole course of my life would change forever.

It wasn't long before the two of us were engaged in a fascinating conversation. It turned out that the old man was a retired British Army officer, who had also served in the diplomatic corps for the Crown. As a result, he had traveled at one time or another to virtually every corner of the globe. And Colonel Bradford, as I shall call him— though it is not his real name—held me spellbound with highly entertaining stories of his adventures.

When we parted, we agreed to meet again, and before long, a close friendship had developed between us. Frequently, we got together at his place or mine for discussions and conversation that lasted late into the night.

On one of these occasions, it became clear to me that

there was something of importance that Colonel Bradford wanted to talk about, but for some reason he was
reluctant to do so. I attempted to tactfully put him at ease,
assuring him that if he wanted to tell me what was on
his mind, I would keep it in strict confidence. Slowly at
first, and then with increasing trust, he began to talk.

While stationed in India some years ago, Colonel Bradford had from time to time come in contact with wander-
ing natives from remote regions of the interior, and he
had heard many fascinating stories of their life and
customs. One strange tale that particularly caught his
interest was repeated quite a number of times, and always
by the natives of a particular district. Those from other
districts seemed never to have heard of it.

It concerned a group of Lamas, or Tibetan priests who,
according to the story, knew the secret of the "Fountain
of Youth." For thousands of years, this extraordinary
secret had been handed down by members of this particular sect. And while they made no effort to conceal it,
their monastery was so remote and isolated, they were
virtually cut off from the outside world.

This monastery and its "Fountain of Youth" had
become something of a legend to the natives who spoke
of it. They told stories of old men who mysteriously
regained health, strength, and vigor after finding and
entering the monastery. But no one seemed to know the
exact location of this strange and marvelous place.

Like so many other men, Colonel Bradford had become
old at the age of 40, and since then had not been growing any younger. The more he heard of this miraculous
"Fountain of Youth," the more he became convinced that
such a place actually existed. He began to gather information on directions, the character of the country, the
climate, and other data that might help him locate the
spot. And once his investigation had begun, the Colonel

became increasingly obsessed with a desire to find this "Fountain of Youth."

The desire, he told me, had become so irresistible, he had decided to return to India and earnestly search for this retreat and its secret of lasting youth. And Colonel Bradford asked me if I would join him in the search.

Normally, I would be the first to be skeptical of such an unlikely story. But the Colonel was completely sincere. And the more he told me of this "Fountain of Youth," the more I became convinced that it could be true. For a while, I was tempted to join the Colonel's search. But as I began to take practical matters into consideration, I finally sided with reason and decided against it.

As soon as Colonel Bradford had left, I began to doubt whether I had made the right decision. To reassure myself, I reasoned that perhaps it is a mistake to want to conquer aging. Perhaps we should all simply resign ourselves to growing old gracefully, and not ask more from life than others expect.

Yet in the back of my mind the haunting possibility remained: a "Fountain of Youth." What a thrilling idea! For his sake, I hoped that the Colonel might find it.

Years passed, and in the press of everyday affairs Colonel Bradford and his "Shangri-La" grew dim in my memory. Then, one evening on returning to my apartment, I found a letter in the Colonel's own handwriting. I quickly opened and read a message that appeared to have been written in joyous desperation. The Colonel said that in spite of frustrating delays and setbacks, he believed that he was actually on the verge of finding "The Fountain of Youth." He gave no return address, but I was relieved to at least know that the Colonel was still alive.

Many more months passed before I heard from him

again. When a second letter finally arrived, my hands almost trembled as I opened it. For a moment I couldn't believe its contents. The news was better than I could possibly have hoped. Not only had the Colonel found "The Fountain of Youth," he was bringing it back to the states with him, and would arrive sometime within the next two months.

Four years had elapsed since I had last seen my old friend. And I began to wonder how he might have changed in that period of time. Had this "Fountain of Youth" enabled him to stop the clock on advancing age? Would he look as he did when I last saw him, or would he appear to be only one year older instead of four?

Eventually the opportunity to answer these questions arrived. While I was at home alone one evening, the house phone rang unexpectedly. When I answered, the door-man announced, "Colonel Bradford is here to see you." A rush of excitement came over me as I said, "Send him right up." Shortly, the bell rang and I threw open the door. But to my disappointment I saw before me not Colonel Bradford, but another much younger man. Noting my surprise, the stranger said, "Weren't you expecting me?"

"I thought it would be someone else," I answered, a little puzzled and confused.

"I thought I would be receiving a more enthusiastic welcome," said the visitor in a friendly voice. "Look closely at my face. Do I need to introduce myself?"

Confusion turned to bewilderment, and then amazed disbelief as I stared at the figure before me. Slowly, I realized that the features of his face did indeed resemble those of Colonel Bradford. But this man looked as the Colonel might have looked years ago in the prime of his life. Instead of a stooping, sallow old man with a cane, I saw a tall, straight figure. His face was robust, and he had a thick growth of dark hair with scarcely a trace of gray.

"It is indeed I," said the Colonel, "and if you don't ask me inside, I'll think your manners badly lacking."

In joyous relief I embraced the Colonel, and unable to contain my excitement, I ushered him in under a barrage of questions.

"Wait, wait," he protested good naturedly. "Allow yourself to catch your breath, and I'll tell you everything that's happened." And this he proceeded to do.

As soon as he arrived in India, the Colonel started directly for the district where the fabled "Fountain of Youth" allegedly existed. Fortunately, he knew quite a bit of the native language, and he spent many months establishing contacts and befriending people. Then he spent many months more putting together the pieces of the puzzle. It was a long, slow process, but persistence finally won him the coveted prize. After a long and perilous expedition into the remote reaches of the Himalayas, he finally found the monastery which, according to legend, held the secret of lasting youth and rejuvenation.

I only wish that time and space permitted me to record all of the things that Colonel Bradford experienced after being admitted to the monastery. Perhaps it is better that I do not, for much of it sounds more like fantasy than fact. The interesting practices of the Lamas, their culture, and their utter indifference to the outside world are hard for Western man to grasp and understand.

In the monastery, older men and women were nowhere to be seen. The Lamas good naturedly referred to the Colonel as "The Ancient One," for it had been a very long time since they had seen anyone who looked as old as he. To them, he was a most novel sight.

"For the first two weeks after I arrived," said the Colonel, "I was like a fish out of water. I marveled at everything

I saw, and at times could hardly believe what was before my eyes. Soon, my health began to improve. I was able to sleep soundly at night, and every morning I awoke feeling more and more refreshed and energetic. Before long, I found that I needed my cane only when hiking in the mountains.

"One morning after I arrived, I got the biggest surprise of my life. I had entered for the first time a large, well-ordered room in the monastery, one that was used as a kind of library for ancient manuscripts. At one end of the room was a full-length mirror. Because I had traveled for the past two years in this remote and primitive region, I had not in all that time seen my reflection in a mirror. So, with some curiosity I stepped before the glass.

"I stared at the image in front of me with disbelief. My physical appearance had changed so dramatically that I looked fully 15 years younger than my age. For so many years I had dared hope that 'The Fountain of Youth' might truly exist. Now, before my very eyes was physical proof of its reality.

"Words cannot describe the joy and elation which I felt. In the weeks and months ahead, my appearance continued to improve, and the change became increasingly apparent to all who knew me. Before long, my honorary title, 'The Ancient One,' was heard no more."

At this point, the Colonel was interrupted by a knock at the door. I opened it to admit a couple who, though they were good friends of mine, had picked this inopportune moment to visit. Concealing my disappointment as best I could, I introduced them to the Colonel, and we all chatted together for a while. Then, the Colonel rose and said, "I am sorry that I must leave so early, but I have another commitment this evening. I hope I shall see all of you again soon." But at the door he turned to me, and said softly, "Could you have lunch with me tomorrow? I promise, if you do, you'll hear all about 'The Fountain of Youth.' "

We agreed to a time and place, and the Colonel departed. As I returned to my friends, one of them remarked, "He certainly is a fascinating man, but he looks awfully young to be retired from army service."

"How old do you think he is?" I asked.

"Well, he doesn't look forty," answered my guest, "but from the conversation I would gather he's at least that old."

"Yes, at least," I said evasively. And then I steered the conversation to another topic. I wasn't about to repeat the Colonel's incredible story, at least not until he had fully explained everything.

The next day, after having lunch together, the Colonel and I went up to his room in a nearby hotel. And there at last he told me full details on "The Fountain of Youth."

"The first important thing I was taught after entering the monastery," said the Colonel, "was this: the body has seven energy centers which in English could be called vortexes. The Hindus call them chakras. They are powerful electrical fields, invisible to the eye, but quite real nonetheless. Each of these seven vortexes centers on one of the seven ductless glands in the body's endocrine system, and it functions in stimulating the gland's hormonal output. It is these hormones which regulate all of the body's functions, including the process of aging.

"The lowest, or first vortex centers on the reproductive glands. The second vortex centers on the pancreas in the abdominal region. The third centers on the adrenal gland in the solar plexus region. The fourth vortex centers on the thymus gland in the chest or heart region. The fifth centers on the thyroid gland in the neck. The sixth

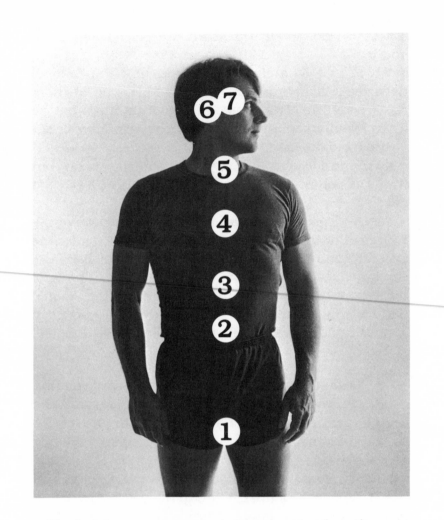

The body's seven energy vortexes are centered on the seven endocrine glands: (1) the reproductive glands, (2) the pancreas, (3) the adrenal gland, (4) the thymus gland, (5) the thyroid gland, (6) the pineal gland, and (7) the pituitary gland.

These energy vortexes revolve at great speed. When all are revolving at high speed, and at the same rate of speed, the body is in perfect health. When one or more of them slow down, aging and physical deterioration set in.

centers on the pineal gland at the rear base of the brain. And the seventh, highest vortex centers on the pituitary gland at the forward base of the brain.*

"In a healthy body, each of these vortexes revolves at great speed, permitting vital life energy, also called 'prana' or 'etheric energy,' to flow upward through the endocrine system. But if one or more of these vortexes begins to slow down, the flow of vital life energy is inhibited or blocked, and—well, that's just another name for aging and ill health.

"These spinning vortexes extend outward from the flesh in a healthy individual, but in the old, weak, and sickly they hardly reach the surface. The quickest way to regain youth, health, and vitality is to start these energy centers spinning normally again. There are five simple exercises that will accomplish this. Any one of them alone is helpful, but all five are required to get best results. These five exercises are not really exercises at all. The Lamas call them 'rites,' and so that is how I shall refer to them too."

RITE NUMBER ONE

"The first rite," continued the Colonel, "is a simple one. It is done for the express purpose of speeding up the vortexes. Children do it all the time when they're playing.

"All that you do is stand erect with arms outstretched, horizontal to the floor. Now, spin around until you become

---

*While there are said to be many, perhaps even thousands of these chakras or vortexes throughout the body, the generally accepted view is that there are seven primary ones. In the original edition of his book Mr. Kelder asserts that one of these is located in the area of the knees. He does not link the vortexes to the endocrine glands. I have taken the liberty of changing this to conform to the more widely held view described here. —*Editor*

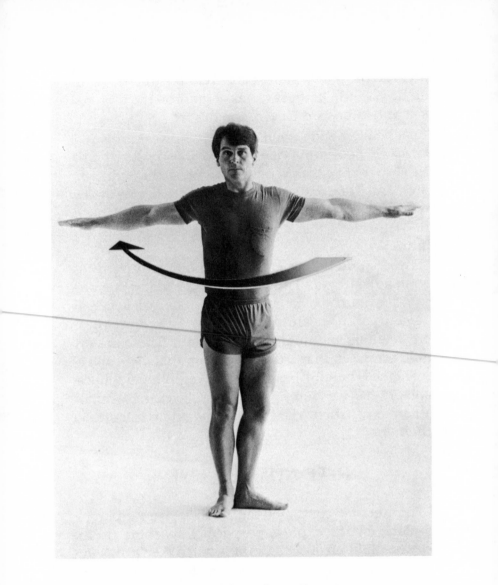

Rite Number 1

slightly dizzy. One thing is important: you must spin from left to right. In other words, if you were to put a clock on the floor face-up, you would turn in the same direction as the clock hands.

"At first, most adults will be able to spin around only about half a dozen times before becoming quite dizzy. As a beginner, you shouldn't attempt to do more. And if you feel like sitting or lying down to recover from the dizziness, then by all means you should do just that. I certainly did at first. To begin with, practice the rite only to the point of slight dizziness. But with time, as you practice all five rites, you will be able to spin more and more times with less dizziness.

"Also, in order to lessen dizziness, you can do what dancers and figure skaters do. Before you begin to spin, focus your vision on a single point straight ahead. As you begin to turn, continue holding your vision on that point as long as possible. Eventually, you will have to let it leave your field of vision, so that your head can spin on around with the rest of your body. As this happens, turn your head around very quickly, and refocus on your point as soon as you can. This reference point enables you to become less disoriented and dizzy.

"When I was in India, it amazed me to see the Maulawiyah, or as they are more commonly known, the whirling dervishes, almost unceasingly spin around and around in a religious frenzy. After being introduced to rite number one, I recalled two things in connection with this practice. First, the whirling dervishes always spun in one direction, from left to right, or clockwise. Second, the older dervishes were virile, strong, and robust. Far more so than most men of their age.

"When I spoke to one of the Lamas about this, he informed me that this whirling movement of the dervishes did have a very beneficial effect, but also a devastating one. He explained that their excessive spinning over-stimulates some of the vortexes, so that they are finally exhausted. This has the effect of first accelerating the flow of vital life energy, and then blocking it. This building up and tearing down action causes the dervishes to experience a kind of 'psychic rush,' which they mistake for something spiritual or religious.

"However," continued the Colonel, "the Lamas do not carry the whirling to excess. While the whirling dervishes may spin around hundreds of times, the Lamas do it only about a dozen times or so, just enough to stimulate the vortexes into action."

RITE NUMBER TWO

"Following rite number one," continued the Colonel, "is a second rite which further stimulates the seven vortexes. It is even simpler to do. In rite number two, one first lies flat on the floor, face up. It's best to lie on a thick carpet or some sort of padded surface. The Lamas perform the rites on what Westerners call a prayer rug, about two feet wide and six feet long. It's fairly thick, and is made from wool and a kind of vegetable fiber. It is solely for the purpose of insulating the body from the cold floor. Nevertheless, religious significance is attached to everything the Lamas do, and hence the name 'prayer rug.'

"Once you have stretched out flat on your back, fully extend your arms along your sides, and place the palms of your hands against the floor, keeping the fingers close together. Then, raise your head off the floor, tucking the chin against the chest. As you do this, lift your legs, knees straight, into a vertical position. If possible, let the legs extend back over the body, toward the head; but do

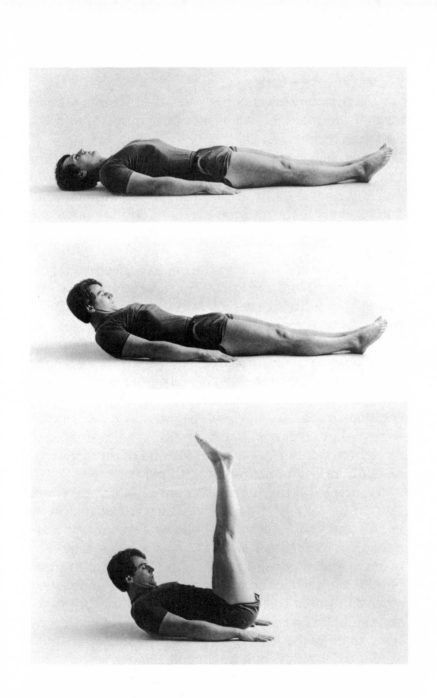

Rite Number 2

not let the knees bend.

"Then, slowly lower both the head and the legs, knees straight, to the floor. Allow all of the muscles to relax, and then repeat the rite.

"With each repetition, establish a breathing rhythm: breathe in deeply as you lift the legs and head; breathe out fully as you lower them. Between repetitions, while you're allowing the muscles to relax, continue breathing in the same rhythm. The more deeply you breathe, the better.

"If you are unable to keep the knees perfectly straight, then let them bend as much as necessary. But as you continue to perform the rite, attempt to straighten them as much as you possibly can.

"One of the Lamas told me that when he first attempted to practice this simple rite, he was so old, weak, and decrepit that he couldn't possibly lift his legs into a straight position. So he started by lifting his legs in a bent position so that his knees were straight up and his feet were hanging down. Little by little, he was able to straighten out his legs until at the end of three months he could raise them straight with perfect ease.

"I marveled at this particular Lama," said the Colonel. "When he told me this, he was the perfect picture of health and youth, although I knew he was many years older than I. For the sheer joy of exerting himself, he used to carry a load of vegetables weighing fully a hundred pounds on his back from the garden to the monastery several hundred feet above. He took his time, but never once stopped on the way up. When he arrived, he didn't seem to be in the least exhausted. The first time that I attempted to follow him up the hill, I had to stop at least a dozen times to catch my breath. Later, I was able to climb the hill as easily as he, and without my cane. But that is another story."

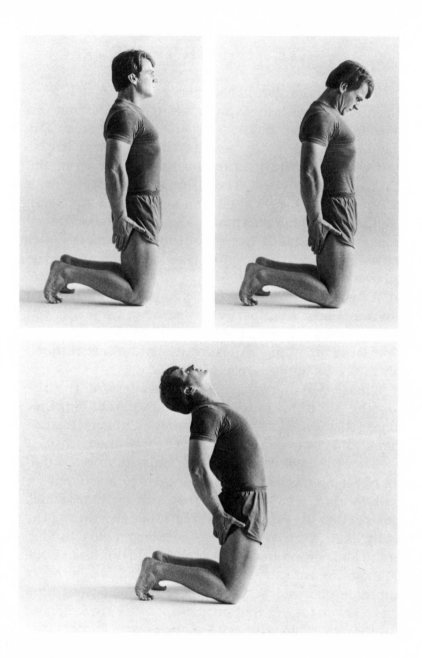

Rite Number 3

RITE NUMBER THREE

"The third rite should be practiced immediately after rite number two. It too is a very simple one. All that you need to do is kneel on the floor with the body erect. The hands should be placed against the thigh muscles.

"Now, incline the head and neck forward, tucking the chin against the chest. Then, throw the head and neck back as far as they will go, and at the same time lean backward, arching the spine. As you arch, you will brace your arms and hands against the thighs for support. After arching, return to the original position, and start the rite all over again.

"As with rite number two, you should establish a rhythmic breathing pattern. Breathe in deeply as you arch the spine. Breathe out as you return to an erect position. Deep breathing is most beneficial, so take as much air into your lungs as you possibly can.

"I have seen more than 200 Lamas perform this rite together. In order to turn their attention within, they closed their eyes. In this manner they eliminated distractions, and could focus themselves inwardly.

"Thousands of years ago, the Lamas discovered that all of the answers to life's imponderable mysteries are found within. They discovered that all of the things which go together to create our lives originate within the individual. Western man has never been able to understand and comprehend this concept. He thinks, as I did, that our lives are shaped by the uncontrollable forces of the material world. For example, most Westerners think it is a law of nature that our bodies must grow old and deteriorate. By looking within, the Lamas know this to be a self-fulfilling illusion.

"The Lamas, especially those at this particular monastery, are performing a great work for the world. It is performed, however, on the astral plane. From this plane, they assist mankind around the globe, for it is high above the vibrations of the physical world, and is a powerful focal point where much can be accomplished with little loss of effort.

"One day the world will awaken in amazement to see the result of great works performed by these Lamas and other unseen forces. The time is fast approaching when a new age will dawn, and a new world will be seen. It will be a time when man learns to liberate the powerful inner forces at his command to overcome war and pestilence, hatred and bitterness.

"So-called 'civilized' mankind is in truth living in the darkest of dark ages. However, we are being prepared for better and more glorious things. Each one of us who strives to raise his or her consciousness to higher levels helps to elevate the consciousness of mankind as a whole. So, performing the five rites has an impact far beyond the physical benefits which they achieve."

RITE NUMBER FOUR

"The first time I performed rite number four," said the Colonel, "it seemed very difficult. But after a week, it was as simple to do as any of the others.

"First, sit down on the floor with your legs straight out in front of you and your feet about 12 inches apart. With the trunk of the body erect, place the palms of your hands on the floor alongside the buttocks. Then, tuck the chin forward against the chest.

"Now, drop the head backward as far as it will go. At the same time, raise your body so that the knees bend while the arms remain straight. The trunk of the body will be in a straight line with the upper legs, horizontal

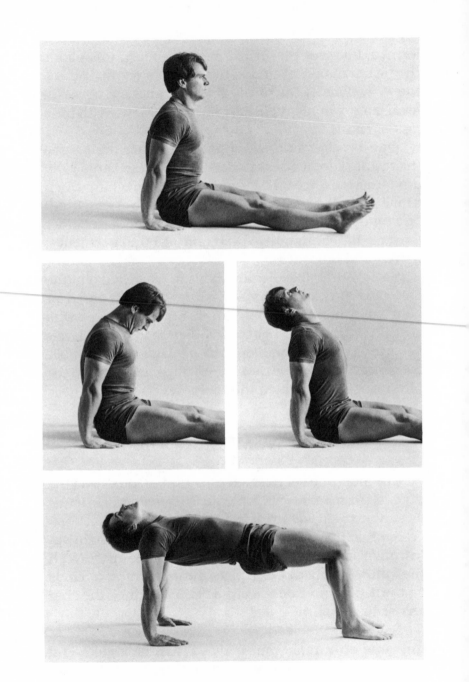

Rite Number 4

to the floor. And both the arms and lower legs will be straight up and down, perpendicular to the floor. Then, tense every muscle in the body. Finally, relax your muscles as you return to the original sitting position, and rest before repeating the procedure.

"Again, breathing is important to this rite. Breathe in deeply as you raise up the body. Hold in your breath as you tense the muscles. And breathe out completely as you come down. Continue breathing in the same rhythm as long as you rest between repetitions.

"After leaving the monastery," continued Colonel Bradford, "I went to a number of larger cities in India, and as an experiment I conducted classes for both English speaking people and Indians. I found that the older members of either group felt that unless they could perform this rite perfectly from the very start, no good could come of it. It was extremely difficult to convince them that they were wrong. Finally, I persuaded them to do the best they could just to see what might happen in a month's time. Once I got them to simply do their best in attempting the rites, the results in one month's time were more than gratifying.

"I remember that in one city I had quite a few elderly people in one of my classes. In attempting this particular rite—number four—they could just barely get their bodies off the floor; they couldn't come close to reaching a horizontal position. In the same class, there were some much younger persons who had no difficulty performing the rite perfectly the very first day. This so discouraged the older people that I had to separate the two groups. I explained to the older group that when I first attempted this rite, I couldn't perform it any better than they. But, I told them, I can now perform 50 repetitions of the rite without feeling the slightest nervous or muscular strain. And to prove it, I did it right before their eyes. From then on, the older group broke all records for progress.

"The only difference between youth and vigor, and old age and poor health is simply the rate of speed at which the vortexes are spinning. Normalize the rate of speed, and the old man becomes like new again."

RITE NUMBER FIVE

The Colonel went on, "When you perform the fifth rite, your body will be face-down to the floor. It will be supported by the hands, palms down against the floor, and the toes in a flexed position. Throughout this rite, the hands and feet should each be spaced about two feet apart, and the arms and legs should be kept straight.

"Start with your arms perpendicular to the floor, and the spine arched, so that the body is in a sagging position. Now, throw the head back as far as possible. Then, bending at the hips, bring the body up into an inverted 'V'. At the same time, bring the chin forward, tucking it against the chest. That's all there is to it. Return to the original position, and start the rite all over again.

"By the end of the first week, the average person will find this rite one of the easiest to perform. Once you become proficient at it, let the body drop from the raised position to a point almost, but not quite, touching the floor. Tense the muscles for a moment both at the raised point, and at the low point.

"Follow the same deep breathing pattern used in the previous rites. Breathe in deeply as you raise the body. Breathe out fully as you lower it.

"Everywhere I go," continued the Colonel, "people at first call these rites isometric exercises. It's true that the five rites are helpful in stretching stiff muscles and joints,

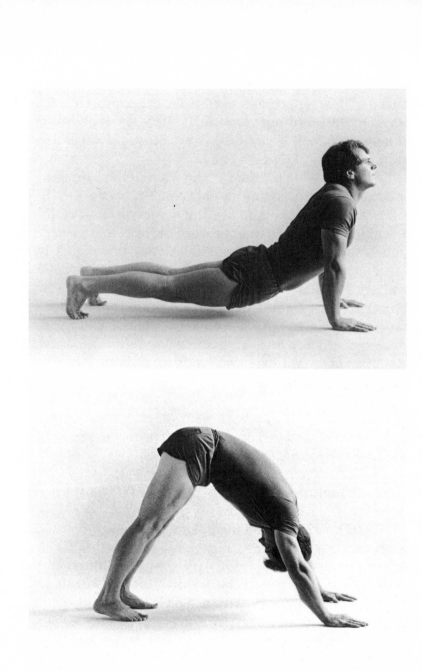

Rite Number 5

and improving muscle tone. But that is not their primary purpose. The real benefit of the rites is to normalize the speed of the spinning vortexes. It starts them spinning at a speed which is right for, say, a strong and healthy man or woman 25 years of age.

"In such a person," the Colonel explained, "all of the vortexes are spinning at the same rate of speed. On the other hand, if you could see the seven vortexes of the average middle-aged man or woman, you would notice right away that some of them had slowed down greatly. All of them would be spinning at a different rate of speed, and none of them would be working together in harmony. The slower ones would be causing that part of the body to deteriorate, while the faster ones would be causing nervousness, anxiety, and exhaustion. So, it is the abnormal condition of the vortexes that produces abnormal health, deterioration, and old age."

A s the Colonel was describing the five rites, questions were popping into my mind. And now that he was finished, I began to ask a few.

"How many times is each rite performed?" was my first question.

"To start with," replied the Colonel, "I suggest that you practice each rite three times a day for the first week. Then every week that follows, increase the daily repetitions by two, until you are performing each rite 21 times a day. In other words, the second week, perform each rite five times; the third week, perform each rite seven times; the fourth week, perform each rite nine times daily, and so on. In ten weeks' time, you'll be doing the full number of 21 rites per day.

"If you have difficulty practicing the first rite, the whirling one, as many times as you do the others, then simply do it as many times as you can without getting too dizzy. Eventually you'll be able to whirl around the full 21 times.

"I knew a man who performed the rites more than a year before he could spin around that many times. He had no difficulty in performing the other four rites, so he increased the spinning very gradually, until he was doing the full 21. And he got splendid results.

"There are a few people who find it difficult to spin around at all. Usually, if they omit the spinning, and perform the other four rites for four to six months, they find that they can then start to handle the spinning too."

"What time of day should the rites be performed?" was my next question to the Colonel.

"They can be performed either in the morning, or at night," he answered, "whichever is more convenient. I perform them both morning and night, but I would not advise so much stimulation for the beginner. After you have been practicing the rites for about four months, you might start performing them the full number of times in the morning, and then at night perform just three repetitions of each rite. Gradually increase these, as you did before, until you are performing the full 21. But it isn't necessary to perform the rites more than 21 times either morning or night, unless you are truly motivated to do so."

"Is each of these rites equally important?" I asked next.

"The five rites work hand-in-hand with each other, and all are equally important," said the Colonel. "After performing the rites for a while, if you find that you are not able to do all of them the required number of times, try splitting the rites into two sessions, one in the morning, and one in the evening. If you find it impossible to do one of the rites at all, omit it and do the other four. Then, after a period of months, try the one you were having difficulty with again. Results may come a little more slowly this way, but they will come nevertheless.

"Under no circumstances should you ever strain yourself. That would be counterproductive. Simply do as much as you can handle, and build up gradually. And never be discouraged. With time and patience there are very few people who cannot eventually perform all five rites 21 times a day.

"In attempting to overcome a difficulty with one of the rites, some people become very inventive. An old fellow in India found it impossible to properly perform rite number four even once. He wouldn't be satisfied with just getting his body off the floor. He was determined that his torso should reach a horizontal position such as I described earlier. So he got a box about ten inches high, and padded the top of it. Then, he lay down flat upon the box, placing his feet on the floor at one end, and his hands on the floor at the other. From this position, he was able to raise his torso to a horizontal position quite nicely.

"Now, this gimmick may not have enabled the old gentleman to perform the rite the full 21 times. But it did make it possible for him to raise his body as high as much stronger men were able to. And this had a positive psychological effect, which in itself was quite beneficial. I do not particularly recommend his technique, but it could help others who think it's impossible to make progress any other way. If you have an inventive mind, you'll be able to think of other ways and means to help yourself perform any rite that may be particularly difficult for you."

Following up on my last question, I asked, "What if one of the rites were left out entirely?"

"These rites are so powerful," said the Colonel, "that if one were left out while the other four were practiced regularly the full number of times, excellent results would still be experienced. Even one rite alone will do wonders, as the whirling dervishes, whom I spoke of earlier, demonstrate. The older dervishes, who did not spin around so excessively as the younger ones, were strong and virile—a good indication that just one rite can have powerful effects. So, if you find that you simply cannot perform all of the rites, or that you cannot perform them the full 21 times, be assured that you will get good results from whatever you are able to do."

I next asked, "Can the rites be performed in conjunction with other exercise programs, or would the two conflict?"

"By all means," said the Colonel, "if you already have some kind of exercise program, continue it. If you don't, then think about starting one. Any form of exercise, but especially cardiovascular exercise, helps the body maintain a youthful equilibrium. In addition, the five rites will help to normalize the spinning vortexes so that the body becomes even more receptive to the benefits of exercise."

"Does anything else go with the five rites," I asked.

"There are two more things which would help. I've already mentioned deep rhythmic breathing while resting between repetitions of the rites. In addition, between each of the rites, it would be helpful to stand erect with your hands on your hips, breathing deeply and rhythmically several times. As you breathe out, imagine that any tension which may be in your body is draining away, allowing you to feel quite relaxed and at ease. As you breathe in, imagine that you are filling yourself with a sense of well-being and fulfillment.

"The other suggestion is to take either a tepid bath or a cool, but not a cold one after practicing the rites. Going over the body quickly with a wet towel, and then with a dry one is probably even better. One thing I must caution you against: you must never take a shower, tub, or wet towel bath which is cold enough to chill you internally. If you do, you will have undone all of the good you have gained from performing the rites."

I was excited at all the Colonel had told me, but deep down inside there must have been some lingering skepticism. "Is it possible that the 'Fountain of Youth' is really as simple as what you have described to me?" I asked.

"All that is required," answered the Colonel, "is to practice the five rites three times a day to begin with, and to gradually increase until you are performing each one 21 times a day. That is the wonderfully simple secret that could benefit all the world if it were known."

"Of course," he added, "you must practice the rites every day in order to achieve real benefits. You may skip one day a week, but never more than that. And if you allow a business trip or some other commitment to interrupt this daily routine, your overall progress will suffer.

"Fortunately, most people who begin the five rites find it not only easy, but also enjoyable and rewarding to perform them every day, especially when they begin to see the benefits. After all, it takes only twenty minutes or so to do all five. And a physically fit person can perform the rites in ten minutes or less. If you have trouble finding even that much spare time, then just get up a few minutes earlier in the morning, or go to bed a little later at night.

"The five rites are for the express purpose of restoring health and youthful vitality to the body. Other factors help determine whether you will dramatically transform your physical appearance, as I have done. Two of these are mental attitude and desire.

"You've noticed that some people look old at 40, while others look young at 60. Mental attitude is what makes the difference. If you are able to see yourself as young, in spite of your age, others will see you that way too. Once I began practicing the rites, I made an effort to erase from my mind the image of myself as a feeble old man. Instead,

I fixed in my mind the image of myself when I was in the prime of life. And I put energy in the form of very strong desire behind that image. The result is what you see now.

"For many people this would be a difficult feat, because they find it impossible to change the way they see themselves. They believe the body is programmed to sooner or later become old and feeble, and nothing will shake them from that view. In spite of this, once they begin to practice the five rites they will begin to feel younger and more energetic. This will help them to change the way they see themselves. Little by little, they will begin to see themselves as younger. And before long, others will be commenting that they have a younger appearance.

"There is one other extremely important factor for those who want to look dramatically younger. There is an additional rite which I've intentionally been holding back on. But rite number six is a subject which I'll save for a later time."

Part Two

No man is free who is a slave to the flesh.
—Lucius Annaeus Seneca

I t had been almost three months since Colonel Bradford's return from India, and a great deal had happened in that time. I had immediately begun practicing
the five rites, and was greatly pleased with the excellent
results. The Colonel had been away tending to personal
matters, so I had been out of contact with him for some
time. When he finally phoned me up again, I eagerly told
him all about my progress, and I assured him that I had
already demonstrated to my complete satisfaction how
very effective the rites can be.

In fact, I had become so enthusiastic about the rites,
I was eager to pass the information on to others who
might also benefit. So I asked the Colonel if he would consider leading a class. He agreed that it was a good idea,
and said that he would do it, but only on three conditions.

The first condition was that the class must contain a
cross section of men and women from all walks of life:
professionals, blue collar workers, homemakers, and so
on. The second condition was that no member of the class
could be under 50 years of age, though they could be a

hundred or more if I could find anyone that old willing to participate. The Colonel insisted on this, even though the five rites are equally beneficial to younger people. And the third condition was that the class be limited to fifteen members. This came as a considerable disappointment to me, because I had envisioned a much larger group. After trying without success to persuade the Colonel to change his mind, I agreed to all three conditions.

Before long, I had managed to assemble a group that met all of the requirements, and right from the beginning the class was a huge success. We met once a week, and as early as the second week I thought that I could see signs of improvement in several of its members. However, the Colonel had asked us not to discuss our progress with one another, and I had no way of knowing whether the others would agree. Then, at the end of the month my uncertainty was put to rest. We held a kind of testimonial meeting at which all of us were invited to share our results. Everyone present reported at least some improvement. Some had glowing accounts of progress, and a few of these could even be called remarkable. A man nearing 75 had made more gains than any of the others.

Weekly meetings of the "Himalaya Club," as we named it, continued. When the tenth week finally came, practically all of the members were performing all of the five rites 21 times a day. All claimed not only to be feeling better, they also believed that they were looking younger, and several even joked that they were no longer telling their real ages. This reminded me that when we had asked the Colonel his age some weeks back, he had said that he would hold that information until the end of the tenth week. Well, the time had arrived, but as yet the Colonel hadn't put in an appearance. Someone suggested that each of us guess the Colonel's age, and write it on a slip of paper. Then, when the truth was announced, we could see who came closest. We agreed to do this, and the slips of paper were being collected as Colonel Bradford walked in.

When we explained what we were up to, Colonel Bradford said, "Bring them here so I can see how well you've done. And then I'll tell you what my age really is." In an amused voice, the Colonel read each of the slips aloud. Everyone had guessed him to be in his forties, and most had guessed the early forties.

"Ladies and gentlemen," he said, "thank you for your very generous compliments. And since you've been honest with me, I'll be the same with you. I shall be 73 years of age on my next birthday."

At first, everyone stared at him in disbelief. Was it really possible for a 73 year old man to look nearly half his age? Then, it occurred to them to ask, why had the Colonel achieved results so much more dramatic than their own?

"In the first place," the Colonel explained, "you have been doing this wonderful work for only ten weeks. When you have been at it two years, you will see a much more pronounced change. But there's more to it than just that. I haven't told you all that there is to know.

"I have given you five rites which are for the purpose of restoring youthful health and vitality. They will also help you regain a younger appearance. But if you really want to completely restore the health and appearance of youth, there is a sixth rite which you must practice. I've said nothing about it up until now, because it would have been useless to you without having first obtained good results from the other five."

The Colonel warned them that in order to take advantage of this sixth rite, they would have to accept a very difficult self-restraint. He suggested that they take some time to consider whether they were willing to do this for the rest of their lives. And he invited those who wished to go on with rite number six to return the following week. After thinking it over, only five of the group came back, though the Colonel said this was a better showing than he had experienced with any of his classes in India.

When he had told them about this additional rite, the Colonel had made it clear that it would lift up the body's reproductive energy. This lifting up process would cause not only the mind to be renewed, but the entire body as well. But he warned that this would entail a restriction which most people were unwilling to accept. Now the Colonel continued with this explanation.

"In the average man or women, part—often a large part—of the vital life force that feeds the seven vortexes is channeled into reproductive energy. So much of it is dissipated in the first vortex that it never has a chance to reach the other six.

"In order to become a superman or superwoman, this powerful life force must be conserved and turned upward, so that it can be utilized by all of the vortexes, especially the seventh. In other words, it is necessary to become celibate so that reproductive energy can be re-channeled to a higher use.

"Now, turning vital life force upward is a very simple matter, and yet, through the centuries, man in attempting it usually fails. In the West, whole religious orders have tried this very thing and failed, because they sought to master reproductive energy by suppressing it. There is only one way to master this powerful urge, and that is not by dissipating or suppressing it, but by *transmuting* it—transmuting it, and at the same time lifting it upward. In this way, you have not only discovered the 'Elixir of Life,' as the ancients called it, you have also put it to use, which is something the ancients were seldom able to do.

"Now, rite number six is the easiest thing in the world

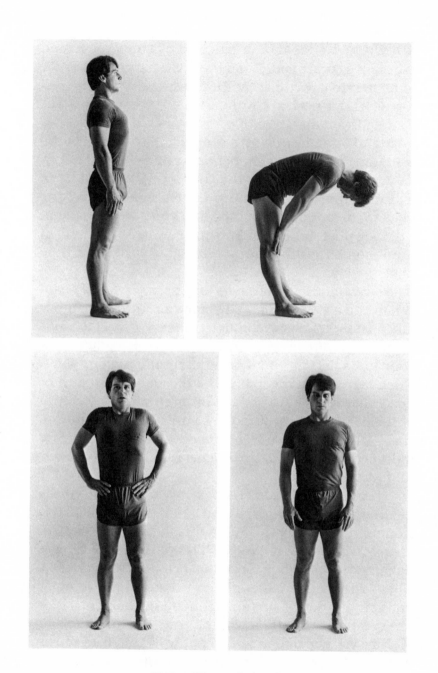

Rite Number 6

to perform. It should be practiced only when you feel an excess of sexual energy, and there is a natural desire for its expression. Fortunately, this rite is so simple that you can do it anywhere, at any time, whenever the urge is felt. Here's all you do:

"Stand straight up and slowly let all of the air out of your lungs. As you do this, bend over and put your hands on your knees. Force out the last trace of air, and then, with the lungs empty, return to a straight up posture. Place your hands on your hips, and press down on them. This will push your shoulders up. As you do this, pull in the abdomen as much as possible, and at the same time raise the chest.

"Now, hold this position as long as you possibly can. When you are finally forced to take air into your empty lungs, let the air flow in through the nose. When the lungs are full, exhale through the mouth. As you exhale, relax your arms, letting them hang naturally at your sides. Then take several deep breaths through the mouth or nose, allowing them to escape through either the mouth or nose. This constitutes one complete performance of rite number six. About three repetitions are required for most people to redirect sexual energy, and turn its powerful force upward.

"There is only one difference between a person who is healthy and vital, and one who is a superman or superwoman. The former channels vital life force into sexual energy, while the latter turns this force upward to create balance and harmony through all of the seven vortexes. That's why a superman or superwoman grows younger and younger day-by-day and moment-by-moment. He or she creates within themself the true 'Elixir of Life.'

"Now you can understand that the 'Fountain of Youth' was within me all the time. The five rites—or six to be more precise—were merely a key that unlocked the door.

When I recall Ponce de Leon and his futile search for 'The Fountain of Youth,' I think what a pity it was that he journeyed so far in order to come up empty handed. He could have achieved his goal without ever leaving home. But like me, he believed that the 'Fountain of Youth' must be in some distant corner of the world. He never suspected that all the time it was right within himself.

"Please understand that in order to perform rite number six, it is absolutely necessary that an individual have active sexual urge. He or she could not possibly transmute reproductive energy if there were little or nothing to transmute. It is absolutely impossible for a person who has lost sexual urge to perform this rite. He or she should not even attempt it, because it would only lead to discouragement, and more harm than good. Instead, such an individual, regardless of age, should first practice the other five rites until they regain a normal sexual urge. When this is achieved, he or she may then go into the business of being a superman or superwoman.

"Also, an individual should not attempt rite number six unless he or she is genuinely motivated to do so. If an individual feels incomplete in terms of sexual expression, and must struggle to overcome its attraction, then that individual is not truly capable of transmuting reproductive energy and directing it upward. Instead, energy will be misdirected into struggle and inner conflict. The sixth rite is only for those who feel sexually complete, and who have a real desire to move on to different goals.

"For the great majority of people, a celibate life is simply not a feasible choice, and they should perform the first five rites only. However, in time the five rites may lead to a changing in priorities, and a genuine desire to become a superman or superwoman. At that time, the individual should make a firm decision to begin a new way of life.

Such an individual must be ready to move forward without wavering or looking back. Those who are capable of this are on their way to becoming true masters, able to use vital life force to achieve anything they desire.

"I repeat, let no man or woman think of turning sexual currents upward until he or she is prepared to leave physical needs behind in exchange for the rewards of true mastership. Then, let that individual step forward, and success will crown his or her every effort."

Part Three

To lengthen thy life, lessen thy meals.
—Benjamin Franklin

A fter the tenth week, Colonel Bradford no longer attended each meeting, but did keep up his interest in the "Himalaya Club." From time to time, he would speak to the group on various helpful subjects, and occasionally members of the group asked advice on something in particular. For example, several of us were especially interested in diet and the tremendously important role that food plays in our lives. There were differing views on the subject, and so we decided to ask Colonel Bradford to describe to us the Lamas' diet, and their policy concerning foods.

"In the Himalayan monastery where I was a neophyte," said the Colonel when he spoke to us the following week, "there are no problems concerning the right foods, nor in getting sufficient quantities of food. Each of the Lamas does his share of work in producing what is needed. All the work is done in the most primitive way. Even the soil is spaded by hand. Of course, the Lamas could use oxen and plows if they wished, but they prefer direct contact with the soil. They feel that handling and working the soil adds something to man's existence. I personally found it to be a thoroughly rewarding experience. It contributed to a feeling of oneness with nature.

"Now, it is true that the Lamas are vegetarians, but not strictly so. They do use eggs, butter, and cheese in quantities sufficient to serve certain functions of the brain, body, and nervous system. However, they do not eat flesh, for the Lamas, who are strong and healthy, and who practice rite number six, seem to have no need of meat, fish, or fowl.

"Like myself, most of those who joined the ranks of the Lamas were men of the world who knew little about proper food and diet. But not long after coming to the monastery, they invariably began to show wonderful signs of physical improvement. And this was due in part at least to their diet there.

"No Lama is choosey about what he eats. He can't be, because there is little to choose from. A Lama's diet consists of good, wholesome food, but as a rule it consists of only one item of food at a meal. That in itself is an important secret of health. When one eats just one kind of food at a time, there can be no clashing of foods in the stomach. Foods clash in the stomach because starches do not mix well with proteins. For example, if bread, which is a starch, is eaten with proteins such as meats, eggs, or cheese, a chemical reaction is set up in the stomach. It not only can cause gas and immediate physical distress. Over time, it also contributes to a shortened life span, and a lesser quality of life.

"Many times in the monastery dining hall I sat down to the table along with the Lamas, and ate a meal consisting only of bread. At other times, we ate nothing but fresh vegetables and fruits. At other meals, I ate nothing but cooked vegetables and fruits.

"At first, I was hungry for my usual diet, and the variety of foods which I had been accustomed to; but before long, I could eat and enjoy a meal consisting of nothing but dark bread, or just one kind of fruit. Sometimes, a meal of just one vegetable would seem like a feast.

"Now, I'm not suggesting that you limit yourself to a diet of just one kind of food per meal, or even that you eliminate meats from your diet. But I would recommend that you keep starches, fruits, and vegetables separate from meats, fish, and fowl at your meals. It is alright to make a meal of just meat. In fact, if you wish, you could have several kinds of meat in one meal. And it is alright to eat butter, eggs, and cheese with a meat meal, or dark bread and, if you wish, coffee or tea. But you must not end up with anything sweet or starchy—no pies, cakes, or puddings.

"Butter seems to be a neutral. It can be eaten with either a starchy meal, or with a meat meal. Milk agrees better with starches. Coffee and tea should always be taken black, never with cream, although a small amount of sweetening will do no harm.

"The proper use of eggs was another interesting and useful thing I learned during my stay in the monastery. The Lamas would not eat whole eggs unless they had been performing hard manual labor. Then, they might eat one whole medium boiled egg. But they would frequently eat raw egg yolks, discarding the whites. At first, it seemed to me to be a waste of perfectly good food to throw the whites to the chickens. But then I learned that the egg whites are utilized only by the muscles, and should not be eaten unless the muscles are exercised.

"I had always known that egg yolks are nutritious, but I learned of their true value only after talking with another Westerner at the monastery, a man who had a background in biochemistry. He told me that common hen eggs contain fully half of the elements required by the brain, nerves, and organs of the body. It is true that these elements are needed only in small quantities, but they must be included in the diet if you are to be exceptionally robust and healthy, both mentally and physically.

"There is one more very important thing which I learned from the Lamas. They taught me the importance of eating slowly, not for the sake of good table manners, but for the purpose of masticating my food more thoroughly. Mastication is the first important step in breaking down food so that it can be assimilated by the body. Everything one eats should be digested in the mouth before it is digested in the stomach. If you gulp down food, bypassing this vital step, it is literally dynamite when it reaches the stomach.

"Protein foods such as meat, fish, and fowl require less mastication than complex starches. It is just as well to chew them thoroughly anyway. The more completely food is masticated, the more nourishing it will be. This means that if you thoroughly chew your food, the amount you eat can be reduced, often by one half.

"Many things which I had taken for granted before entering the monastery seemed shocking when I left it two years later. One of the first things I noticed when I arrived in one of the major cities of India was the large amount of food consumed by everyone who could afford to do so. I saw one man eat in just one meal a quantity of food sufficient to feed and completely nourish four hard working Lamas. But of course the Lamas would never dream of putting into their stomachs the combinations of food which this man consumed.

"The conglomeration of foods in one meal was another thing that appalled me. Having been in the habit of eating one or two foods at a meal, I was amazed to count 23 varieties of food one evening at my host's table. No wonder Westerners have such miserable health. They seem to know little or nothing about the relation of diet to health and strength.

"The right foods, the right combinations of food, the right amounts of food, and the right method of eating combine to produce wonderful results. If you are over-weight, it will help you to reduce. And if you are under-weight, it will help you to gain. There are quite a few other points about food and diet that I would like to go into, but time doesn't permit. Just keep in mind these five things:

(1) Never eat starch and meat at the same meal, though if you are strong and healthy, it need not cause you too much concern now.
(2) If coffee bothers you, drink it black, using no milk or cream. If it still bothers you, eliminate it from your diet.
(3) Chew your food to a liquid, and cut down on the amount of food you eat.
(4) Eat raw egg yolks* once a day, every day. Take them either just before or after meals—not during the meal.
(5) Reduce the variety of foods you eat in one meal to a minimum."

*The U.S.D.A. recommends against the consumption of raw eggs which can be contaminated with salmonella bacteria. —*Editor*

Part Four

Colonel Bradford was addressing the "Himalaya Club" for the last time before leaving to travel to other parts of the U.S. and his native England. He had chosen to speak on various things other than the five rites which help in the rejuvenation process. And as he stood before the group, he appeared to be sharper, more alert, and more vigorous than ever before. Immediately after his return from India, he had seemed to be the image of perfection. But since then, he had continued to improve, and even now he was making new gains.

"First of all," said the Colonel, "I must apologize to the women in our group, because much of what I have to say tonight will be directed to the men. Of course, the five rites which I have taught you are equally beneficial to men and women. But being a man myself, I would like to speak on a subject of importance to other men.

"I'll begin by talking about the male voice. Do you know that some experts can tell how much sexual vitality a man has just by listening to him speak? We have all heard the shrill, piping voice of a man who is advanced in age.

Unfortunately, when an older person's voice begins to take on that pitch, it's a sure sign that physical deterioration is well under way. Let me explain.

"The fifth vortex at the base of the neck governs the vocal cords, and it also has a direct connection with the first vortex in the body's sexual center. Of course, all of the vortexes have common connections, but these two are, in a manner of speaking, geared together. What affects one affects the other. As a result, when a man's voice is high and shrill, it's an indicator that his sexual vitality is low. And if energy in this first vortex is low, you can bet that it's lacking in the other six as well.

"Now, all that's necessary to speed up the first and fifth vortexes, along with all the others, is to practice the five rites. But there is another method which men can use to help speed up the process. It's easy to do. All that's required is willpower. You simply need to consciously make the effort to lower your voice. Listen to yourself speak, and if you hear yourself becoming higher or more shrill, adjust your voice to a lower register. Listen to men who have good, firm speaking voices, and take note of the sound. Then, whenever you speak, keep your voice down in that masculine pitch as much as possible.

"A very old person will find this to be quite a challenge, but the reward is that it does bring excellent results. Before long, the lowered vibration of your voice will speed up the vortex in the base of the throat. That, in turn, will help speed up the vortex in the sexual center, which is the body's doorway to vital life energy. As the upward flow of this energy increases, the throat vortex will speed up still more, helping the voice to go still lower, and so on.

"There are young men who appear to be robust and virile now, but who, unfortunately, will not remain that way for long. That is because their voices never fully matured, and remained rather high. These individuals, as well as the older ones I've been talking about, can get wonderful results by consciously making the effort to lower their voices. In a younger person, this will help to preserve virility, while in the older one it will help to renew it.

"Sometime ago I came across an excellent voice exercise. Like other effective things, it is quite simple. Whenever you are by yourself, or where there is sufficient noise to drown your voice so you won't disturb others, practice saying in a low tone, partly through the nose, 'Mimm—Mimm—Mimm—Mimm.' Repeat it again and again, lowering your voice in steps, until you've forced it as low as you possibly can. It's effective to do this first thing in the morning when the voice already tends to be in a lower register. Then, make an effort to hold your voice in a low pitch for the rest of the day.

"Once you start making progress, practice in the bathroom so you can hear your voice reverberate. Then,try to get the same effect in a larger room. When the vibration of your voice is intensified, it will cause the other vortexes in the body to speed up, especially the first one in the sexual center, and the sixth and seventh in the head.

"In older women, the voice can also become high and shrill, and it should be toned down in this same manner. Of course, a woman's voice is naturally higher than a man's, and women should not attempt to lower their voices to the point of sounding masculine. In fact, it would be beneficial for a woman whose voice is abnormally masculine to attempt to raise her voice pitch, using the method already described.

"The Lamas chant in unison, sometimes for hours, in a low register. The significance of this is not the chanting itself, or the meaning of their words. It is the vibration of their voices and its effect on the seven vortexes.

Thousands of years ago, the Lamas discovered that the vibratory rate of the sound 'Oh-mmm . . .' is especially powerful and effective. Both men and women will find it highly beneficial to chant this sound at least several times each morning. It's still more helpful to repeat it again throughout the day whenever you can.

"Fill your lungs completely with air, and standing erect, slowly expel the full breath to create one 'Oh-mmm . . .' sound. Divide it roughly half and half between the 'Ohhh . . .' and the 'Mmmm . . . .' Feel the 'Ohhh. . .' vibrate through the chest cavities and the 'Mmmm . . .' vibrate through the nasal cavities. This simple exercise helps greatly to align all of the seven vortexes, and you'll be able to feel its benefits almost right from the very start. Don't forget, it is the vibration of the voice that is significant, not the act of chanting, or the meaning of the sound.

"Now," said the Colonel, after pausing a moment, "everything I've taught you so far has concerned the seven vortexes. But I'd now like to discuss a few things that can make us all much younger, even though they do not directly affect the vortexes.

"If it were possible to suddenly take an aging man or woman out of a decrepit old body and place them in a young, new one about 25 years of age, I'd be willing to bet that he or she would continue to act old, and to hold onto the attitudes that helped make them old in the first place.

"Though most people will complain about advancing age, the truth is they get a dubious pleasure out of growing old and all the handicaps that come with it. Needless to say, this attitude isn't going to make them any younger. If an older person truly wants to grow younger, they must think, act, and behave like a younger person, and eliminate the attitudes and mannerisms of old age.

"The first thing to pay attention to is your posture.

Straighten up! When you first started this class, some of you were so bent over that you looked like question marks. But as vitality began returning, and your spirits improved, your posture improved also. That was fine, but don't stop now. Think about your posture as you go about your daily activities. Straighten your back, throw your chest out, pull in your chin, and hold your head high. Right away you have eliminated 20 years from your appearance, and 40 years from your behavior.

"Also, get rid of the mannerisms of old age. When you walk, know first where you are going; then start out and go directly there. Don't shuffle; pick up your feet and stride. Keep one eye on the place where you're going, and the other on everything you pass.

"At the Himalayan monastery there was a man, like myself a Westerner, whom you would have sworn was not over 35 years of age, and who acted like a man of 25. He was actually more than a hundred years old. If I told you how much over a hundred, you wouldn't believe me.

"In order for you to achieve this kind of miracle, you must first desire to do so. You must then accept the idea that it is not only probable, but certain that you will. As long as the goal of growing younger is an impossible dream to you, it will remain just that. But once you fully embrace the wonderful reality that you can indeed become younger in appearance, health, and attitude, and once you energize that reality with focused desire, you have already taken your first drink of the healing waters of the 'Fountain of Youth.'

"The five simple rites which I have taught you are a tool or a device that can enable you to achieve your own personal miracle. After all, it is the simple things of life which are most powerful and effective. If you continue to perform these rites to the best of your ability, you will be ever so richly rewarded.

"It has been most gratifying to see each of you improve from day to day," concluded the Colonel. "I have taught you all that I can for the present. But as the five rites continue to do their work, they will open doors to further learning and progress in the future. In the meantime, there are others who need the information which I have taught you, and it is time for me to be on my way to them."

At this the Colonel bade us all farewell. This extraordinary man had earned a very special place in our hearts, and so of course, we were sorry to see him go. But we were also glad to know that before long others would be sharing the priceless information which he had so generously given us. We considered ourselves fortunate indeed. For in all of history, few have been privileged to learn the ancient secret of the "Fountain of Youth."

PUBLISHER'S NOTE

If you practice the five rites, we welcome you to write to us with comments on your experiences. Address letters to: Harbor Press, P.O. Box 1656, Gig Harbor, WA 98335.

Peter Kelder's book is the only source known to us for information on the author or the five rites per se. We regret that we are unable to furnish additional details.